Essential Oil Recipes:

Enhance Your Health, Beauty, and Home

By John Gordon

Table of Contents

Introduction 5

Chapter 1: Household Essential Oil Recipes 6

Chapter 2: Essential Oil Diffuser Recipes/Mixtures 18

Chapter 3: Gift Ideas Using Essential Oil Recipes 31

Chapter 4: Essential Oil Beauty Product Recipes 41

Chapter 5: Essential Oil Food Recipes 53

Conclusion 64

written consent and can in no way be considered an endorsement from the trademark holder.

Introduction

Congratulations on purchasing this book on essential oil recipes and thank you for doing so.

The following chapters will discuss the many ways that one can use essential oils. With the recent popularity of essential oil diffusers, it is easy to overlook the numerous other methods that can employ the usage of these wonderful oils.

This book contains many recipes for essential oils and how you can use them in your day-to-day life. You will find ways to use essential oils in cooking, making blends for diffusers, making essential oil candles, creative gifts with essential oils, and much more. Detailed instructions for each recipe will be provided, as well as any other information you might need to get the full effect of each recipe.

Essential oils are so popular because of their many uses and benefits. We will explore the benefits of essential oils along with their many uses so that you are fully aware of what each product can do for you. Some examples of benefits of using essential oils are how they can improve digestion, help to relax the body and muscles, soothe pains and cramps, and to relieve headaches. These are just a few of the countless benefits, which we will delve further into within this book!

There are plenty of books on the subject of essential oils on the market, thanks again for choosing this one! Every effort was made to ensure it is full of as much useful information as possible, please enjoy!

Chapter 1: Household Essential Oil Recipes

Improving your everyday household items has never been easier! There are many ways to use essential oils to improve your cleaning products, carpet cleaners, laundry products, and more.

This chapter will provide a multitude of recipes for your home that use essential oils. Soon you will not want to use your normal household products without essential oils at all!

Homemade Essential Oil Fabric Softener

This recipe will take just minutes to prepare and will leave your clothes smelling fresh and feeling soft!

The recipe below uses Castile soap, which is a soap product made exclusively of vegetable oils. This type of soap is commonplace in most stores, including Walmart and Walgreens. You can also order it online if you do not feel like going to the store to get it!

Items you need:
- Lavender essential oil: 4-5 drops
- Vinegar, white: 0.33 Cups
- Baking soda: 0.5 Cups
- Bergamot essential oil: 4-5 drops
- Castile soap (Lavender scented works great with this recipe): 0.25 Cups

How to make it:
- Mix the drops of essential oils and the Castile soap into your normal soap dispenser of a loaded washing machine

- Pour in the baking soda over the clothes that are in the washing machine
- Add the white vinegar into the dispenser for fabric softener. You may also add this in during the final rinse cycle of the washing machine if you choose to do so
- Turn the washing machine on the appropriate temperature settings as you normally would
- Finish the wash and move clothes to the dryer to enjoy your wonderfully scented fabrics!

Dryer Sheets made with Essential Oils

Dryer sheets add a wonderful smell to clothing items, towels, and other fabrics. This recipe to make your own dryer sheets will improve the smell even more and will add a touch of essential oil to your fabrics so that you can reap the benefits of essential oils just by wearing your everyday clothes!

Items you need:
- Vinegar, white: 1 Cup
- Lemongrass essential oil: 9-10 drops
- Lavender essential oil: 9-10 drops
- Color-resistant (colorfast) fabric, previously washed: 3 feet
- Jar, large: 1

How to make it:
- Rip or cut the color-resistant fabric into 24 squares
- Place the fabric squares into the large jar and add in the drops of both essential oil scents
- Add the white vinegar into the jar and mix the liquids in with the fabrics until each square is evenly coated
- Use 1 dryer sheet for 1 load of laundry as you normally would. Enjoy the wonderful scents left on your fabric!

Makeup Brush Essential Oil Cleaning Liquid

Cleaning your makeup brushes with this recipe will offer a new-like bristle on each brush! It will also help to add essential oils to your makeup so that you feel its benefits on your skin in a subtle way. With this, you can make your skin healthier than ever as it absorbs the essential oils!

This recipe is best to use at least once a week for the fullest effect!

Items you need:
- Lemon essential oil drops: 1-2
- Tea Tree essential oil drops: 2-3
- Castile liquid soap, unscented: 1 t

How to make it:
- Place the oils and liquid soap into the palm of one of your hands
- Mix a dampened makeup brush into the oil and soap mixture on your hand and swirl around so that the brush is coated in the liquid
- Wipe off the excess liquid stuck to the brush with your fingers and run it under water for a few seconds
- Allow the brush to dry on a paper towel for a few hours
- Once dry, use the makeup brush as you normally would!

Essential Oil Wipes for Cleaning

You can wipe down your counters and leave behind the wonderful scent of essential oils with this recipe. Making these everyday wipes is incredibly easy and will not take you much time at all!

You can get any liquid cleaner you prefer for this recipe, although it should be unscented.

Items you need:
* Jar, large: 1
* Liquid cleaner: 0.5 t
* Eucalyptus essential oil: 9-10 drops
* Tea tree essential oil: 9-10 drops
* Lemon essential oil: 9-10 drops
* Vinegar, white: 0.25 Cups
* Water: 0.75 Cups
* 3-ply napkins: 20-25

How to make it:
* In the jar, mix together all of the essential oils, the vinegar, water, and liquid cleanser
* Place the napkins into the jar and turn the jar until each napkin has been evenly coated with the liquid
* Use when necessary and keep the wipes in a dry place with a secured lid on the jar!

Essential Oil Dish Soap

This recipe will give you the familiar bubbly suds to clean dishes that you are used to, but made from your own home! You will leave healthy essential oils on dishes to get a better clean and will not use nearly as many harsh chemicals compared to store-bought dish soap!

For the dispenser for the soap, you can use an old, cleaned out soap or cleaner dispenser. Otherwise, you can certainly find a new dispenser at the store. Just make sure it has a pump for you to use!

Items you need:
- Dispenser with pump: 1
- Basil essential oil: 3-4 drops
- Lemon essential oil: 6-7 drops
- Liquid cleaner: 0.25 Cups
- Water: 1.5 Cups

How to make it:
- Mix the essential oil drops and the water in the glass jar
- Put the liquid cleaner into the jar with the essential oil and water and mix together
- Spray on dishes or into warm water as needed!

Essential Oil Shower Cleaner

This easy-to-make shower cleaner does not require scrubbing! Not only will your shower smell wonderful after each use, cleaning it is made even easier. Just spray this cleaner after your shower onto the walls and door and let it sit for 3-4 minutes before rinsing it off.

The thieves essential oil used in this recipe is somewhat uncommon. The thieves smell is a combination of lemon, cinnamon, clove, rosemary, and eucalyptus. You can purchase this form of essential oil online at sites like Amazon, or you could mix your own. If this is undesirable as well, you could substitute this oil for a preferred essential oil scent.

Items you need:
- Thieves essential oil: 11-12 drops
- Liquid cleaner: 1.5 t
- Vinegar, white: 1 Cup
- Water: 1 Cup
- Tea tree essential oil: 9-10 drops
- Spray bottle: 1

How to make it:
- Place the vinegar and water into the dispenser and mix them together
- Add in the essential oil drops and liquid cleaner to the vinegar and water mixture and combine all of the ingredients
- Place the sprayer lid onto the filled dispenser and use as needed

---

Essential Oil Insect Repellant

The smell of store-bought bug sprays is usually not very pleasant. Well, this recipe will change that! You will love the smell of this homemade insect repellant, and you will love how it keeps bugs off of you when you are enjoying the outdoors.

Items you need:
- Aloe Vera gel: 4 oz.
- Grapefruit essential oil: 5 drops
- Lemongrass essential oil: 2 drops
- Thyme essential oil: 3 drops
- Jasmine essential oil: 3 drops
- Spray bottle: 1 container

How to make it:
- Pour the Aloe Vera gel into the spray bottle
- Add the essential oil drops into the gel-filled spray bottle and stir all of the ingredients together
- Spray on your skin lightly when needed or spray around doors and entrance ways to your home to prevent bugs from getting in!

Essential Oil Toilet Cleaner

This *essential* household item is simple to make with *essential* oils! Just spray this product into your toilet bowl at night and let it sit while you sleep. In the morning, scrub the toilet with a brush and flush!

Items you need:
- Borax: 0.25 Cups
- Vinegar, white: 1 Cup
- Baking soda: 0.25 Cups
- Lemon essential oil: 6 droplets
- Tea tree essential oil: 6 droplets
- Medium bowl: 1

How to make it:
- Place the borax, vinegar, baking soda, and essential oil drops into the bowl
- Stir the ingredients together to combine
- Pour the mixture into your toilet when ready to use!

Tile Cleaner with Essential Oils

Mopping your tile floors has never smelled so wonderful! For this recipe, you should mix all of the ingredients together and then add them to a full pail of water. Then mop as you normally would!

Items you need:
- Pine essential oil: 18 drops
- Peppermint essential oil: 12 drops
- Orange essential oil: 12 drops
- Vinegar, white: 1 Cup
- Baking soda: 0.25 Cups
- Bowl, small: 1

How to make it:
- Mix the essential oil drops, vinegar, and baking soda in the bowl
- When ready to mop, put the essential oil mixture into the pail of water and soak the mop!

Multi-Surface Essential Oil Scrub

Rid yourself of those hard to get spots and clean like you never have before! This multipurpose scrubbing agent will make your home have a lovely fragrance and will clean it perfectly.

Items you need:
- Large bowl: 1
- Vinegar, white: 1 T
- Baking soda: 1 Cup
- Castile liquid soap: 3 T
- Pine essential oil: 8 drops
- Peppermint essential oil: 13 drops
- Lemon essential oil: 9 drops

How to make it:
- Place the soap, essential oil drops, vinegar, and baking soda into the bowl and mix together
- Scrub the mixture on dirty surfaces as needed and dry

Carpet Essential Oil Deodorizer

Shake this recipe onto your carpet for a wonderful scent that will last for days! Not only will it improve the smell of your carpet, but it will help clean it too!

The shaker bottle used in this recipe can be bought at Walmart or online. It should be similar to a parmesan cheese shaker that you would see in a restaurant for improved shaking power!

Purification essential oil is a combination of many different scents. If you cannot find it online or in stores, you can use a combination of other scents you have on hand to substitute.

Items you need:
- Shaker bottle: 1
- Purification essential oil: 15 drops
- Baking soda: 1 Cup

How to make it:
- Put the drops of essential oils and all of the baking soda into the glass shaker
- Stir the oil and baking soda together until they are well mixed
- Place the lid on the shaker and sprinkle over your carpet
- Let the deodorizer set for 10 minutes before vacuuming over as usual

---

Essential Oil "Poo-Pourri" Spray

You may have seen the sprays to get rid of bad toilet odor, but now you can make your own! This recipe is sure to smell even better than the store-bought versions so that you never have to worry about a stinky bathroom again.

For the vegetable glycerin in this recipe, you can purchase it online or in stores. Most convenience stores carry this product, as well as most hobby/craft stores.

*You may also want to have a funnel to pour the ingredients into the spray bottle depending on what items you have handy

Items you need:
- Eucalyptus essential oil: 14 drops

- Peppermint essential oil: 12 drops
- Lemongrass essential oil: 14 drops
- Vegetable glycerin: 1 t
- Water: 0.5 Cups
- Plastic spray bottle: 1
- Small bowl: 1

How to make it:
- Place the essential oil drops, vegetable glycerin, and water into the bowl
- Combine the ingredients in the bowl and then pour into the spray bottle
- Spray the essential oil spray around your toilet prior to going to the bathroom and enjoy the lovely scent!

Essential Oil Oven Cleaner

It happens to just about everyone, we use our ovens over and over without cleaning them, and soon enough the grime is caked on. This dirt can seem impossible to get off, but not with this essential oil cleaner! Your oven will look brand new and smell better than ever before.

Items you need:
- Water: 0.25 Cups
- Baking soda: 0.75 Cups
- Tea tree essential oil: 12 drops
- Pine essential oil: 14 drops
- Orange essential oil: 14-15 drops
- Bowl, small: 1

How to make it:
- Mix the essential oil drops and the baking soda in the small bowl

- Add the water to the small bowl and combine together well until a paste-like substance has shaped. Use more water if there are chunks of baking soda still present
- Dampen a cloth and use it to wipe down a completely cooled oven with essential oil cleaner
- Let the cleaner sit in the oven for about 5 minutes before removing and wiping down

---

Essential Oil Detergent Pods

You may not think that you cannot make your own pods for the dishwashing machine, but it is certainly possible! This recipe makes the pods to add to your dirty dishes and uses essential oils to make your dishes smell great and get a full-on clean.

You will need a silicone mold for this recipe, preferably one that is split up into squares. You can purchase this item at most stores. Be sure that each square is the right size to fit in the pod holder of your dishwasher.

Items you need:
- Water: 0.5 Cups
- Citrus essential oil: 45 drops
- Salt: 3 T
- Arm & Hammer Super Washing Soda: 1.25 Cups
- Square silicone mold: 1
- Bowl, small: 1

How to make it:
- Place the essential oil drops, water, washing soda, and salt into the bowl and combine them well
- Scoop an even amount of the mixture into each silicone mold square and pat each one down
- Let the filled mold sit to dry for 24-48 hours

- Pop out the pods once they are all dry and store in an air-tight container
- Use one pod at a time and put into your dishwasher as you normally would

The recipes previously provided in this chapter are sure to make your home fresher than it has ever been. These cleaning items will enhance your home and fill it with the wonderful smells of essential oils.

Get ready to experiment in creative ways with your essential oils and love your home more in the process!

Chapter 2: Essential Oil Diffuser Recipes/Mixtures

Most people are aware that essential oils can be used for diffusers, and they have certainly grown in popularity over recent years. Who wouldn't want their homes to smell wonderful and give off healthful aromas?

This chapter will provide many essential oil diffuser mixtures to try. Sometimes it can be hard to find new combinations of essential oils to diffuse, but this chapter is sure to assist you with this.

Motivating Tanger-Clove

The combination of essential oils in this recipe will help motivate you to perform any task you wish. Mixing the scents of this diffuser recipe will rejuvenate you and make you want to get work done!

Items you need:
- Ginger essential oil: 3 drops
- Tangerine essential oil: 1 drop
- Clove essential oil: 2 drops

Chai Spice

Chai is a lovely smell that can relax and improve the mood of anyone around it. This diffuser combination will smell of chai and will be accompanied by all of the benefits of it as well.

The cassia essential oil used in this recipe is similar to cinnamon, but with even more benefits. Cassia is known for its anti-depressant pain-relieving qualities, which will further enhance this diffuser mixture.

Items you need:
- Clove essential oil: 3 drops
- Ginger essential oil: 2 drops
- Cardamom essential oil: 2 drops
- Cassia essential oil: 1 drop

Fall Walk

The combination of essential oils in this mixture forms an immune system boosting formula. Using this diffuser mixture when the illness is going around is a great idea to help prevent it from getting to you. The fragrance will also remind you of a mid-fall day, making the experience of it even better.

Items you need:
- Cinnamon bark essential oil: 3 drops
- Wild orange essential oil: 2 drops
- Eucalyptus essential oil: 2 drops
- Clove essential oil: 2 drops
- Rosemary essential oil: 2 drops

Sleepytime Oils

You may have heard of "Sleepytime Tea", but now you can have it in your diffuser. These oils combine into a relaxing scent that will help you fall asleep in no time! Great for those restless nights that make sleeping seem impossible.

The Vetiver essential oil in this recipe comes from a fragrant grass-like plant known for its antiseptic properties. Mixing it in with the other essential oils of this recipe improve upon the benefits of all the oils!

Items you need:
- Vetiver essential oil: 4 drops
- Chamomile essential oil: 1 drop
- Lavender essential oil: 1 drop

Better than my Husband's Cologne

Do not tell the men in your life, but this diffuser recipe is better than the cologne that they use! The masculine smell of this recipe isn't just for men to enjoy though, as everyone is sure to love it. The woodsy hints of it are fit for everyone and are sure to fill the room with happy men and women.

Items you need:
- Cypress essential oil: 1 drop
- Wintergreen essential oil: 2 drops
- White fir essential oil: 4 drops

Calm and Warm Blend

This recipe is great for when you desire a relaxing afternoon. The essential oil combination has decompressing effects that let you take it easy and take the night off!

Items you need:
- Cedarwood essential oil: 2 drop2
- Pine essential oil: 1 drop
- Frankincense essential oil: 3 drops

Herb and Citrus

Mixing herbs and citrus produces a lovely taste in food and will create and even better scent in your diffuser. This combination might inspire you to cook more fragrant meals, but it is also sure to please with scent alone!

Items you need:
- Marjoram essential oil: 3 drops
- Lemon essential oil: 3 drops
- Basil essential oil: 2 drops

Juice and Joy

This mood-boosting recipe can lighten your mood and please your senses. The grapefruit smell blends well with the other scents to make you happy all day long!

The Joy essential oil used in this recipe is best known for its quality that increases feelings of comfort and bliss. The smell of this oil is a combination of floral and citrus scents, including lemon, jasmine, and rose.

Items you need:
- Grapefruit essential oil: 2 drops
- Joy essential oil: 4 drops

Stone Sour

This recipe would surely be a sour one in the fruit's original forms! In the essential oils, though, you can fill your home with the clean citrus scent that you are sure to love!

Items you need:
- Wild orange essential oil: 2 drops
- Lime essential oil: 2 drops
- Lemon essential oil: 4 drops
- Grapefruit essential oil: 2 drops

Odor Be Gone

Face it, accidents happen. Sometimes those accidents leave an odor behind even after it is cleaned up that is hard to get rid of. This recipe of essential oils can cover up and get rid of unwanted smells in your home while leaving a new, fresh smell in its place.

Did you know that tea tree is also referred to as Melaleuca? The name Melaleuca refers to the plant that the tea tree oil is extracted from, so the two names are often used interchangeably. This oil is known for medicinal properties, especially in terms of skin care health.

Items you need:
- Lime essential oil: 2 drops
- Cilantro essential oil: 1 drop
- Tea tree essential oil: 2 drops
- Lemon essential oil: 3 drops

Fresh Flower

The calming scent of flowers is strong with this recipe. Who needs a bouquet when you can have this diffuser recipe? The fragrance of it is sure to make you never want to buy real flowers ever again.

Items you need:
- Chamomile essential oil: 3 drops
- Geranium essential oil: 2 drops
- Lavender essential oil: 3 drops

Lovely Mind

This blend of plant oils is meant to help you prepare your mind to focus and be present while enjoying the lovely scents around you. Combining many of the most popular scents has never been so great!

Items you need:
- Lavender essential oil: 3 drops
- Peppermint essential oil: 2 drops
- Rosemary essential oil: 2 drops
- Grapefruit essential oil: 3 drops
- Lemon essential oil: 3 drops
- Basil essential oil: 2 drops

Stress Relief

Many essential oil blends help to alleviate stress, but this one is perfect for those especially rough days. This combination is the perfect formula to help you become less stressed and able to focus on what needs to be done.

The ylang-ylang essential oil in this recipe is derived from a tree of the same name. This oil has grown in popularity over recent years for use in aromatherapy and perfume mixtures. It is especially well known for its ability to lower blood pressure and decrease stress pertaining to the nervous system, making it the perfect addition to this recipe! It can be bought at your favorite essential oil retailer as well.

Items you need:
- Lavender essential oil: 4 drops
- Ylang ylang essential oil: 2 drops
- Marjoram essential oil: 1 drop
- Sage essential oil: 3 drops

Rejuvenate

Blends of powerful scents to fill your home and mind with positive energy! This recipe is great all year round and will impress guests and family members every time.

Items you need:
- Lemon essential oil: 4 drops
- Peppermint essential oil: 4 drops
- Rosemary essential oil: 4 drops

Mint Gum

This blend is reminiscent of your favorite minty chewing gum! Perfect for after dinner to refresh yourself.

Items you need:
- Rosemary essential oil: 2 drops
- Spearmint essential oil: 3 drops
- Peppermint essential oil: 2 drops

Woodsy Nutmeg

This comforting blend is mellow and enjoyable. You will love this combination and smells, especially the boost of nutmeg essential oil in it!

Items you need:
- Citrus essential oil: 2 drops
- Frankincense essential oil: 2 drops
- Nutmeg essential oil: 2 drops

Winter Noon

A scent perfect for winter, but you will want to diffuse it all year long anyway! You will love this blend of winter scents with a hint of lemon.

The Balsam fir essential oil used in this recipe is from the needles of a tree in North America that gives off a woody scent. You have likely seen this tree represented most around the winter time.

Items you need:
- Balsam Fir essential oil: 2 drops
- Lemon essential oil: 2 drops
- Frankincense essential oil: 2 drops

Ready for Christmas

Despite the name, this recipe is great for all holidays all throughout winter time!

The Christmas Spirit essential oil can be bought online or at your favorite essential oil retailer. This oil has a spicy mixture of spruce, cinnamon, and orange. A perfect combination for winter!

Items you need:
- Tangerine essential oil: 4 drops
- Christmas spirit essential oil: 6 drops

Spicy Pepper

Spices, spices, and more spices! The spicy essential oil scents have lovely aromas and make it easier to put your mind and body at ease. This blend is no exception and has a perfect combination of spices to fill your home with.

Items you need:
- Frankincense essential oil: 3 drops
- Black pepper essential oil: 3 drops

Herbal Refresh

Blends with herbs, citrus, and spice to get your home smelling nice! This scent is extremely refreshing and will be a fan favorite in your household in no time.

Items you need:
- Eucalyptus essential oil: 2 drops
- Sage essential oil: 2 drops
- Bergamot essential oil: 2 drops
- Cypress essential oil: 2 drops

Crisp Morning:

Waking up in the morning isn't always easy, but this blend will help you get a jump start. Just get this blend diffusing as soon as possible in the morning, and you are sure to be ready to go in no time.

Items you need:
- Lavender essential oil: 2 drops
- Cypress essential oil: 3 drops
- Tea tree essential oil: 3 drops

Cozy Evening

Warm up your night with this lovely blend. Nothing better than snuggling up under a blanket and reading a good book, which is exactly what this scent will make you want to do!

Items you need:
- Bergamot essential oil: 2 drops
- Ginger essential oil: 2 drops
- Coriander essential oil: 2 drops

Sweater Weather

Put your sweater on for this aroma. It is the perfect scent to enjoy a cold winter day. You will love the woody scent all day long.

Items you need:
- Orange essential oil: 2 drops
- Cedarwood essential oil: 3 drops
- Cardamom essential oil: 2 drops

Peppermint Bark

Your favorite holiday treat can now be your favorite diffuser scent! This blend is strong and will make you crave the candy version as your house smells just like it.

Items you need:
- Peppermint essential oil: 3 drops
- Cinnamon bark essential oil: 2 drops

Sunny Day

This blend is made up of all the sunny-colored oils you could want. It will give your home a refreshing, citrusy scent that will boost your mood and improve your day! Let's do it, sunshine!

Items you need:
- Lemon essential oil: 4 drops
- Bergamot essential oil: 2 drops
- Grapefruit essential oil: 3 drops
- Orange essential oil: 3 drops

Ginger Spice

This blend will remind you of gingerbread cookies baking in a hot oven. The scents will fill your home with the spicy smell of ginger and baked goods so that everyone there will be happy, and maybe even hungry!

Items you need:
- Ginger essential oil: 3 drops
- Cardamom essential oil: 2 drops
- Christmas spirit essential oil: 2 drops

Rose Gold

Your favorite jewelry color made fragrance! The rose smell mixed with the other scents will give your home an effeminate, welcoming aroma for all to enjoy.

Items you need:
- Rose essential oil: 4 drops
- Vanilla essential oil: 2 drops

- Cardamom essential oil: 2 drops

Respiratory Relief

This blend is a mixture to help you achieve healthier lungs. Essential oils are a safe, non-toxic aromatherapy method anyway, but this combination is even better for respiratory support! Breather better and live better with this scent!

Items you need:
- Tea tree essential oil: 3 drops
- Lavender essential oil: 3 drops
- Lemon essential oil: 2 drops

Prairie Day

This blend has a very earthy, comforting scent that will make you want to go outside and lay in the grass. Fill your home with the lovely field smell that everyone will love!

The petitgrain essential oil used in this recipe is derived from the leaves and twigs of an orange tree! The normal orange essential oil typically comes from the peels of an orange, but this oil gives an earthy tone that orange essential oil does not achieve. This oil is known for its antiseptic properties and relaxing effects on the nervous system.

Items you need:
- Petitgrain essential oil: 5 drops
- Jasmine essential oil: 3 drops
- Rosemary essential oil: 3 drops

Diffuser recipes can be boring and repetitive if you always use the same ones. Now you have a large variety of unique recipes to use each and every day that you will never grow tired of!

The blends given in this chapter will help you love your home and love your diffuser every day. You are meant to enjoy life on every occasion, and these recipes will help you to achieve that!

Chapter 3: Gift Ideas Using Essential Oil Recipes

Essential oils themselves are great gifts, but what if you could make them into ready-to-use presents? These recipes are sure to please any gift receiver and will make the holidays fun for everyone.

Whether it is for a secret Santa gift or for an in-law, these crafty ideas are the perfect gift-giving go-to!

Essential Oil Diffusing Ornament

Ornaments are a simple, yet perfectly festive gift to give around the holiday times. This recipe will help you to make your own ornaments to give out that people are sure to love.

You will need to get air-drying clay for this recipe, which is easily purchased at craft stores or online.

Soon your friends will have a wonderful ornament that gives off a lovely scent all season long!

Items you need:
- Parchment paper: Enough to cover the area that you will be making the ornament in
- Air-drying clay: 1 full container
- Rosemary essential oil: 3 drops
- Peppermint essential oil: 3 drops
- Cinnamon bark essential oil: 4 drops
- Clove essential oil: 4 drops
- Ribbon: 8-10 inches worth
- Paintbrush: 1
- Acrylic paint, choice of color: 1 small container
- Holiday cookie cutter: 1
- Rolling pin: 1

How to make it:
- Place the parchment paper over your working space
- Put the clay in your hands and manipulate it until it is warmed and soft
- Roll out the clay with the rolling pin until the clay is about a quarter of an inch thick
- Place the cookie cutter onto the clay and press down. Cut out the shape pressed onto the clay. Repeat this until the rolled out clay is used up. Be sure to cut out a hole somewhere in the clay to put the ribbon through
- Allow the ornament to dry on the parchment paper for 1 day
- Paint the dried ornament on one side with the acrylic paint. Allow to dry
- Pull the ribbon through the ornament and tie it at the end
- Paint on the essential oils mixture to the unpainted side of the ornament. The smell may begin to fade after a week or more, so you can paint on more oils as necessary

---

Perfume with Essential Oils

The perfect stocking stuffer, this perfume is better than any expensive store-bought perfume you could get. Not to mention the essential oil benefits that come along with using it!

The Palo Santo essential oil in this recipe is a great scent. Palo Santo is a type of wood known for its healing properties. Those properties are transferred into this lovely perfume for you to enjoy as well!

Items you need:
- 100 proof vodka: 1.5 t
- Vanilla extract: 0.25 t
- Palo Santo essential oil: 4 drops

- Frankincense essential oil: 6 drops
- Orange essential oil: 11 drops
- Spray bottle: 1 10-ml bottle
- Funnel, small: 1

How to make it:
- With the funnel at the top of the opened spray bottle, pour the essential oil drops, vanilla, and vodka into it
- Place the sprayer back on the bottle securely and shake it until all of the ingredients are combined
- Spray the perfume on as desired

Men's Essential Oil Body Wash

Gifting this body wash is perfect for the men in your life. The essential oils have a masculine scent and help to a get a nice clean feeling! You can put this wash in a decorative bottle of your choice to make it even more festive.
The vitamin E oil and Jojoba oil in this recipe are both plant-based oils that help create healthy skin. The Jojoba oil might be a bit harder for you to find in stores, but can certainly be purchased online. Japanese Cypress essential oil can also be bought online and from your favorite essential oil vendors!

Items you need:
- Bottle with lid: 3 oz. container
- Vitamin E oil: 0.5 t
- Jojoba oil: 0.5 t
- Marjoram essential oil: 4 drops
- Japanese Cypress essential oil: 4 drops
- Castile liquid soap: 3.5 T

How to make it:
- Place the essential oil drops, Jojoba oil, vitamin E oil, and liquid soap into the empty bottle

- Securely put the lid onto the bottle and shake well until the ingredients are completely combined
- Use on normal bathing brushes and enjoy!

Essential Oil Diffusing Necklace

Making jewelry can be tedious and bothersome, but not with this recipe. Not only will the process be fun, but you can also give this lovely gift to others for them to enjoy. The necklace smells wonderful and diffuses the essential oil scents for everyone to take in. This gift is sure to please!

The Hemp cord used in this recipe is perfect for necklaces. You can buy a large quantity of it for a low price on Amazon, but could certainly find it at a craft store as well. You may also use any essential oil scent that you desire. The receiver of this gift will want to add more essential oil to the necklace as the scent fades, usually every other week or so.

Items you need:
- Air-drying clay: 1 full container
- Wax paper
- Rolling pin: 1
- Hemp Cord: 15-20" per necklace depending on how long you want the necklaces to be
- Pen cap: 1
- Small lid: 1 (can be from a soda bottle or any other bottle)
- Stamp: 1 (will put a design on the necklace)
- Japanese Cypress essential oil: 4 drops (or use any preferred scent)

How to make it:
- Lay out the wax paper over the area in which you will be working

- Place the clay onto the wax paper and roll it out flat with the rolling pin until it is about a quarter of an inch thick
- Press the small lid onto the rolled out clay like a cookie cutter and pull out the cut clay that will be your necklace shape
- Use the pen cap to cut out a small hole to run the cord through for your necklace
- Press the stamp lightly onto the prepared necklace piece to form a decorative design
- Allow the necklace to dry for at least 1 day
- Run the hemp cord through the pendant and tie it off at the end
- Spray the essential oil on the outward facing part of the necklace
- Wear and enjoy!

Decorative Essential Oil Disks

Decorative disks made with essential oils will make the perfect gift for any time of the year! Just put these disks in a cute glass bowl and enjoy the wonderful fragrance omitted from them!

Make these disks extra special by using a shaped cookie pan or mold of your choice. There are many options on the market, including flowers and other designs. Just be sure to get a mold or pan that makes the disks about 2 inches wide for the best effect.

Items you need:
- Lavender essential oil: 10-12 drops
- Lemon essential oil: 14-15 drops
- Vanilla extract: 1 T
- Cookie pan or silicone mold: 1
- Water: 0.25 Cups
- Non-stick spray

- Baking soda: 1 Cup
- Glass bowl to put the disks in: 1
- Mixing bowl: 1

How to make it:
- Place the essential oil drops, vanilla, water, and baking soda into the mixing bowl
- Stir the mixing bowl of items together in the bowl until well mixed
- Spray an even coat of the non-stick spray over the cookie pan or mold
- Spoon the mixture into the greased cookie pan or mold in even amounts to make the disks
- Allow the disks to dry in the pan overnight so that they solidify
- Remove the disks from the pan and place into the glass bowl to give out

---

Peppermint Essential Oil Scrub

This holiday-scented scrub is great for use all over your body. It is the perfect gift to give to someone who needs some relaxation in their life and can be extra decorative by using a cute mason jar with lace on it! Feel free to get creative with the packaging of this gift, as it will only add to the wonderful product inside!

Items you need:
- Glass Mason jar: 1 (about 6 oz.)
- Peppermint essential oil: 13 drops
- Avocado oil: 0.25 Cups
- Baking soda: 0.25 Cups
- Sugar: 0.25 Cups
- Mixing bowl: 1

How to make it:
- Place the essential oil drops, avocado oil, baking soda, and sugar into the mixing bowl
- Combine the ingredients in the mixing bowl well
- Scoop the mixture into the mason jar
- Decorate the jar as desired and prepare to gift the wonderful scrub!

Essential Oil Air Freshener Pendants

These cute gifts are great for those that love hanging air fresheners in their car or home! You can just tie these pendants wherever you desire and enjoy the smells. Be sure to have the essential oils reapplied whenever the scent begins to fade!

Items you need:
- Ribbon: enough to tie and hang the pendants
- Scissors
- Parchment paper
- Cypress essential oil: 3 drops
- Idaho Balsam Fir essential oil: 2 drops
- Baking sheet: 1
- Drinking straw: 1
- Rolling pin
- Air drying clay: 1 container (get a colored variety for more fun!)
- Clay cutter, desired shape: 1
- Oven-baking clay: 1 container

How to make it:
- Make sure your oven is heating to 275 degrees Fahrenheit
- Take the oven-baking clay into your hands and work it until it is warmed and softened

- Use the rolling pin to flatten out the oven-baking clay and the air drying clay separately, each to about an eighth of an inch thickness
- Place the air drying clay carefully on top of the oven-baking clay and use the rolling pin again to press out any wrinkles that might have formed
- Press the clay cutters into the formed clay and make as many pendants as desired
- Remove the excess clay from around the cut pieces
- Use the straw to form a hole in each pendant and pull it out. This is where you will run the ribbon through later on
- Cover the baking sheet with parchment paper and then place the clay pendants on it
- Place the baking sheet with pendants into the heated oven and allow it to cook in the oven for 30 minutes
- Take out the baking sheet from the oven and let it to cool completely
- Run the ribbon strands through each pendant and form a loose knot at the end so that it is easily undone for the person that wants to hang it
- Cover 1 side of each pendant with the essential oil drops
- Reapply the essential oils when the scent begins to fade

Homemade Essential Oil Body Butter

Do you know anyone that loves beauty products to enhance their skin? Well then this gift will be perfect for them! Using this body butter made with essential oils will leave your skin smooth and healthy, not to mention the lovely smell. The gift receiver will also love the thoughtfulness of this homemade product.

The Frankincense oil in this recipe can be bought at your favorite essential oil retailer. This essential oil has a wonderfully earthy smell. It is also known for its effects to create radiant skin and enhance your spiritual connections from its earthy tones.

Items you need:
- Coconut Oil: 0.25 Cups
- Shea Butter: 0.75 Cups
- Frankincense essential oil: 10-11 drops
- Vitamin E oil: 1 t
- Glass jar: 1 8 oz. container
- Mixing bowl: 1

How to make it:
- Place the vitamin E oil, shea butter, and coconut oil into the mixing bowl and blend together with a whisk or hand mixer
- Scrape the sides of the bowl and continue to blend until the ingredients have doubled in size
- Put the drops of essential oil into the bowl of blended ingredients and beat the ingredients for 20-30 more seconds
- Scoop the blended mixture into the glass jar and secure it with a lid
- Decorate the jar as desired!

Essential Oil Lip Balm

Looking for another good stocking stuffer or a small, simple gift? Look no further as this lip balm is the perfect choice. The essential oils will help to moisturize and replenish lips so that they are soft healthy. This gift is sure to please!

Items you need:
- Shea butter: 2 t
- Geranium essential oil: 1 drop
- Bergamot essential oil: 2 drops
- Vanilla extract: 0.25 t

- Vitamin E oil: 0.5 t
- Coconut oil: 1 t
- Avocado oil: 1 T
- Double boiler: 1
- Lipstick tube: 1
- Beeswax: 2 t

How to make it:
- Place the coconut oil, vanilla, vitamin E oil, beeswax, avocado oil, and shea butter into the double boiler and mix them together
- Heat the double boiler until the ingredients are melted
- Take the ingredients away from the source of heat and stir in the essential oil drops
- Put the mixture into the lipstick tube and allow it to cool

---

Give lovely gifts with essential oils for all to love! This chapter is full of gifts that others are sure to love. The essential oils in each gift make them special and more beneficial than other, everyday gifts!

Chapter 4: Essential Oil Beauty Product Recipes

So far we have explored a variety of products that you can make with essential oils, all of which are fantastic products! This chapter focuses on beauty products to enhance skin and make you feel refreshed each day.

We have already seen a few beauty product recipes already, but these will be all encompassing! You will love your new skin and clean feelings after using the recipes provided in this chapter.

Honey & Oat Essential Oil Face Scrub

We all know someone that could use a spa day, likely even ourselves! Using this scrub will make anyone feel refreshed and revitalized just like you went to the actual spa. This scrub should be made when you are just about ready to use it so that the essential oils do not dissipate from the scrub.

Items you need:
- Lavender essential oil: 2-3 drops
- Hot water: 1 T
- Buttermilk: 1 T
- Honey: 1 T
- Old-fashioned oats: 0.25 Cups
- Mixing bowl: 1

How to make it:
- Place the essential oil drops, honey, buttermilk, water, and oats into the mixing bowl
- Mix the ingredients in the bowl well until a creamy texture has formed
- Apply the scrub to your face and rinse!

Essential Body Oil

This soothing formula is meant to be used after your shower to make your skin extra soft! It will help moisturize your skin and will give off a lovely scent to go along with it. Just apply to slightly wet skin and enjoy!

Items you need:
- Dropper bottle: 1 1 oz. container
- Avocado oil: 1 oz.
- Geranium essential oil: 2 drops
- Bergamot essential oil: 2 drops
- Chamomile essential oil: 1 drop
- Lavender essential oil: 2 drops
- Jasmin essential oil: 2 drops

How to make it:
- Place the essential oil drops and the avocado oil into the dropper bottle
- Secure the lid onto the dropper oil and shake until the ingredients are well combined
- Swirl bottle before each use to recombine the ingredients

Essential Oil Blemish Remover

It never fails that on an important day you have some form of blemish on your face. Fear not, you can now use the power of essential oils and other beneficial ingredients to remove blemishes in no time!

The calendula gel used in this recipe is a necessary ingredient for relieving irritated skin. This gel is great for burns, bites, and stings, and, of course, blemishes! Combining this with the essential oils and borage oil boosts the impact of this recipe.

You can buy calendula gel and the borage oil online or at Walgreens.

Items you need:
- Lipgloss container: 1
- Eucalyptus essential oil: 1 drop
- Fennel essential oil: 1 drop
- Lemon essential oil: 1 drop
- Tea tree essential oil: 11 drops
- Borage oil: 0.5 t
- Calendula gel: 1.5 t
- Mixing bowl: 1
- Funnel, small: 1

How to make it:
- Place the essential oil drops, borage oil, and calendula gel into the mixing bowl and stir to combine
- Use the funnel to pour the ingredients from the mixing bowl into the lip gloss container. Place the lid securely on the container until ready to use
- Apply the blemish remover to skin where blemishes have formed!

Facial Essential Oil Toner

Cleanse your face with this wonderful facial toner. It is sure to cover up pores and make your skin radiate!

The Witch Hazel used in this recipe might be hard to find in stores. However, you can find it online and on Amazon.com for under $10 for a 16 oz. bottle! This gel is derived from a plant of the same name and is known for its ability to tighten skin and minimizing pores.

Items you need:
- Round cotton pads: 1 packages

- Mason jar: 1 8-oz. jar
- Geranium essential oil: 13 drops
- Lavender essential oil: 2 drops
- Water: 0.5 Cups
- Witch Hazel: 0.5 Cups

How to make it:
- Place the Witch Hazel, water, essential oil drops, and cotton pads into the mason jar
- Secure the mason jar lid onto the jar and shake until all of the liquid is evenly coated on the cotton pads
- Apply one cotton pad to your face when ready to use

Cuticle Rejuvenating Oil

Washing your hands consistently is obviously good for many reasons and can help prevent the spread of disease. However, it can also dry out the cuticles on your nails. Do not worry though, because this product will rehydrate your cuticles for strong, healthy nails!

Items you need:
- Vitamin E oil: 0.5 t
- Avocado oil: 1.5 T
- Lavender essential oil: 20 drops
- Dropper bottle: 1 1-oz. bottle

How to make it:
- Pour the essential oil drops, avocado oil, and vitamin E oil into the dropper bottle
- Secure the lid onto the bottle and shake it until all of the ingredients are well combined
- Drop the oil onto your cuticles and massage until fully absorbed

Essential Oil Overnight Conditioner

The weather and heated products we use on our hair can be damaging, but you can certainly revitalize your hair! This conditioner will repair damaged and brittle hair. Leave it in your hair overnight so that the oils are sufficiently absorbed to improve the texture of your hair and make it smell great. Use this conditioner about once a month or so for the best effect!

Items you need:
- Wintergreen essential oil: 2 drops
- Lavender essential oil: 2 drops
- Sage essential oil: 2 drops
- Jojoba oil: 0.25 t
- Mixing bowl: 1

How to make it:
- Place the essential oil drops and jojoba oil into the mixing bowl and mix well
- Massage the mixture into your hair right away for the best outcome

---

Fresh Mint Mouthwash

Clean out your mouth with this mouthwash that does not burn! That's right, no alcohol in this mouthwash means you get all of the cleanliness of using a normal mouthwash, but without the burn and with plenty of healthy essential oils!

Items you need:
- Container with pour spout: 1 8-oz. container
- Thieves essential oil: 3 drops
- Peppermint essential oil: 4 drops
- Spearmint essential oil: 2 drops
- Baking soda: 1 t
- Water: 1 cup

How to make it:
- Place the essential oil drops, baking soda, and water into the container
- Secure the lid onto the container and shake until the ingredients are combined
- Use this mouthwash daily for best effect!

Ache Away Cream

Many essential oils have the benefit of being muscle relaxers and alleviating joint pain. This cream will use these medical benefits and optimize their usage. Now you can stop any suffering and make your skin healthy in the process!

The Panaway essential oil used in this recipe combines wintergreen, the helichrysum flower, cloves, and peppermint to create a powerhouse of soothing remedies. You can buy this oil at your favorite essential oil retailer or, as always, Amazon!

Items you need:
- Panaway essential oil: 28 drops
- Coconut oil: 0.5 Cups
- Copaiba essential oil: 12 drops
- Glass jar: 1 4-oz. container
- Mixing bowl: 1

How to make it:
- Heat the coconut oil in a microwave until melted, about 5-10 seconds
- Place the essential oil drops and coconut oil into the mixing bowl and stir until well combined
- Pour the mixture into the glass jar and secure the lid on it
- Store the cream in a cool, dark place until it has solidified
- Apply the cream to aching areas of the body and enjoy!

All-Day Leave-In Conditioner

This dry conditioner spray is great to put in damaged hair to leave in all day to help make it healthy. It can repair hair and give you a good hair day on those late start mornings!

Items you need:
- Glass spray bottle: 1 2-oz. container
- Rosemary essential oil: 3 drops
- Frankincense essential oil: 3 drops
- Geranium essential oil: 3 drops
- Lavender essential oil: 3 drops
- Jojoba oil: 0.25 t
- Water: 1 oz.

How to make it:
- Pour the Jojoba oil, water, and essential oil drops into the spray bottle
- Secure the lid onto the spray bottle and shake until the ingredients are well combined
- Spray onto hair as needed and shake the bottle prior to each usage

---

Essential Oil Hair Detangling Spray

You do not want to damage your hair by trying to yank knots out of it. Using this spray will help get those pesky knots out and will only make your hair healthier! You will even get the benefits of the essential oils that are mixed in.

Items you need:
- Spray bottle: 1 2-oz. container
- Avocado oil: 0.25 t
- Lavender essential oil: 12 drops
- Vegetable glycerin: 0.5 t
- Aloe Vera gel: 1 t

- Water: 10 t

How to make it:
- Place the water, avocado oil, Aloe Vera gel, vegetable glycerin, and essential oil drops into the spray bottle container
- Secure the lid onto the spray bottle and shake it until all of the ingredients are well combined
- Spray onto hair in problem areas as needed

Homemade Essential Oil Shampoo

Making your own shampoo is very easy! And this one will add a lot of healthy moisture to your hair and will replenish any damages it might have thanks to the essential oils!

Items you need:
- Tea tree essential oil: 22 drops
- Orange essential oil: 12 drops
- Joy essential oil: 20 drops
- Jojoba oil: 2 t
- Coconut milk, unsweetened: 0.5 Cups
- Fragrance-free shampoo: 1 Cup
- Squeeze bottle: 1 14-oz. bottle

How to make it:
- Place the fragrance-free shampoo, essential oil drops, coconut milk, and jojoba oil into the squeeze bottle
- Secure the lid onto the squeeze bottle and shake until the ingredients are combined. This may take a few minutes to get the shampoo ingredients equally mixed in
- Store the shampoo in the fridge until ready to use and return to the fridge after use

Scalp Rejuvenating Oil

This oil is great to rub on your head and get rid of dead skin cells so that they do not cause any buildup. It will also help to grow long, healthy hair when used regularly. This is partly due to the wonderful essential oils, as well as the nourishing olive oil.

Items you need:
- Cypress essential oil: 1 drop
- Basil essential oil: 1 drop
- Ylang Ylang essential oil: 1 drop
- Lavender essential oil: 1 drop
- Rosemary essential oil: 2 drops
- Olive oil: 2 T
- Mixing bowl: 1

How to make it:
- Place the olive oil and all of the essential oil drops into the mixing bowl
- Combine all the ingredients until well incorporated.
- Apply the oils to your scalp and massage lovingly and let sit for half an hour before rinsing out

---

Essential Oil Hair Rinse

Sometimes the store-bought hair products we use can cause nasty buildup in our hair. It can be hard to get out, but this rinse recipe makes it easy. Get a deep clean on your hair and get a fresh start on creating healthy locks with essential oils. Use weekly for the best effect!

Items you need:
- Water: 1 cup
- Apple cider vinegar: 2 T
- Tea tree essential oil: 1 drop

- Rosemary essential oil: 1 drop
- Lavender essential oil: 1 drop
- Small bowl: 1

How to make it:
- Place the water, apple cider vinegar, and essential oil drops into the small bowl
- Mix the ingredients together until well combined
- Bring the bowl of ingredients into the shower with you to use after shampooing your hair and rinsing it out

---

Homemade Essential Oil Shower Bombs

Get ready to enhance your showering experience with these homemade shower bombs. Just place them on the shower floor with you in an area that is away from a direct water stream and enjoy! You will love the way your shower smells and the effect that it has on your skin from the essential oils!

Items you need:
- Silicone mold: 1 (use any preferred design you want, get ~1 oz. size molds)
- Peppermint essential oil: 120 drops
- Lavender essential oil: 80 drops
- Water: 0.33 Cups
- Cornstarch: 2 T
- Baking soda: 1 Cup
- Mixing bowl: 1

How to make it:
- Make sure your oven is heating to 200 degrees Fahrenheit
- Place the water, cornstarch, and baking soda into the mixing bowl and stir until they are well combined
- Pour about 1 T of the mixture into each hole of your mold

- Place the filled mold into the heated oven and let it bake for 2 hours, or until completely dry
- Remove the mold from the oven and allow to cool. Once cooled, remove each of the bombs from their molds
- Add 7-8 drops of essential oil to each shower bomb, using more peppermint than lavender on each one
- Store until ready to use

Essential Oil Milk Bath

Sometimes it is relaxing to end the day with a simple bath. Now you can make your bath even more relaxing by using this essential oil milk bath mixture. This recipe will only take seconds to prepare so that you are ready to unwind in your bath almost immediately.

Items you need:
- Eucalyptus essential oil: 12 drops
- Cypress essential oil: 8 drops
- Milk, warm: 1 Cup
- Small bowl: 1

How to make it:
- Fill your bathtub with water until a desired amount is in the tub
- Place the essential oil drops and the milk into the bowl and stir together
- Slowly add the essential oils and milk mixture to the bathtub, being sure to stir it into the bathwater as it goes in
- Get in the tub and enjoy!

Using the recipes provided in this chapter will give you a new sense of relaxation and will make you feel better about yourself overall. You will add moisture to your skin and hair, as well as making them both healthier in the process.

Essential oils are a wonderful addition to any beauty product, and now you can add them from home whenever you want!

Chapter 5: Essential Oil Food Recipes

We have seen many of the external benefits of essential oils and how to use them, but did you know that they can safely be consumed as well? Essential oils can help nourish your body and give you more energy to get through your day. They also make a tasty addition to your foods!

Peppermint Essential Oil Fudge

This recipe is great for the holidays, but is still crave-worthy all year round! You will love the peppermint flavor in this sweet treat!

Items you need:
- Parchment paper
- Peppermint essential oil: 12 drops
- Marshmallow crème: 1 7-oz. jar
- Semi-sweet chocolate: 12 oz.
- Sugar: 3 Cups
- Butter: 12 T
- Evaporated milk: 1 5-oz. can
- Baking pan: 1 9x13 inch pan
- Saucepan: 1

How to make it:
- Line the baking pan with parchment paper
- Place the sugar, butter, and evaporated into the saucepan and heat it over medium heat on the stove
- Continuously stir the ingredients in the saucepan until it comes to a boil. Continue to do this until the saucepan ingredients reach 235 degrees Fahrenheit
- Take the saucepan of ingredients away from the heat source

- Add the marshmallow crème and semi-sweet chocolate to the saucepan and stir until they have melted and combined completely with the other ingredients
- Stir in the essential oil drops to the other ingredients
- Pour the saucepan of ingredients into the lined baking pan and allow it to cool completely before cutting

---

Cran-apple Essential Oil French Toast

This sweet breakfast dish is a great way to start your day right. The essential oils are present in the sauce and French toast so that you get full flavors and a satisfyingly full stomach!

Items you need:
- Bread slices: 12
- Ginger essential oil: 1 drop
- Clove essential oil: 2 drops
- Nutmeg essential oil: 1 drop
- Vanilla extract: 1 t
- Butter, melted: 0.5 Cups
- Milk: 0.75 Cups
- Eggs: 3
- Cinnamon bark essential oil: 3 drops
- Orange essential oil: 4 drops
- Apple, chopped: 1 small (a green apple will provide the best flavor)
- Berry preserves: 1 Cup
- Apple juice: 0.5 Cups
- Dried cranberries: 1 Cup
- Saucepan: 1
- Mixing bowl: 1

How to make it:
- Place the apple juice, cranberries, berry preserves, and apples into the saucepan and heat on a low setting until a simmer has formed

- Take the saucepan of ingredients away from the heat and stir in 1 drop of the cinnamon essential oil and 2 drops of the orange essential oil
- Set the saucepan of ingredients aside
- Place a griddle onto a heat source and get it to 375 degrees Fahrenheit
- Place the nutmeg essential oil drops, vanilla, butter, milk, eggs, clove essential oil drop, ginger essential oil drop, and the rest of the orange and cinnamon bark essential oil drops into the mixing bowl
- Whisk the mixing bowl ingredients together and dip each slice of bread into the mixture
- Hold the bread slices over the bowl to allow excess to liquid to come off and then place each slice onto the heated griddle
- Cook each side of the bread for 3-4 minutes or until slightly crisped on each side
- Take the bread slices from the griddle and top with the cranberry and applesauce before eating

---

Essential Oil Dark Chocolate and Orange Candies

Orange and chocolate pair well together. You can now even create this wonderful pairing with the help of essential oils. Not only will the flavor be satisfying, but the essential oils and dark chocolate will add a heart-healthy boost of nourishment!

Items you need:
- Melting chocolate, dark: 1 Cup
- Double boiler: 1
- Candy mold: 1 sheet
- Lollipop sticks: 1 package
- Orange essential oil: 5 drops

How to make it:
- Place the dark chocolate into the double boiler and heat until just melted, being sure to stir as it melts
- Add the orange essential oil drops to the melted chocolate and stir them in
- Pour the chocolate and essential oil mixture into the candy mold immediately so that it does not harden
- Stick the lollipop sticks into each individual chocolate mold and allow the candy to cool completely before removing each piece from the mold

---

Tangy Essential Oil Guacamole

This guacamole is unlike any other! The essential oils give it a tangy twist to add a boost of flavor, while still keeping the favorite tastes of other guacamole recipes. You will get a ton of healthy fats in this tasty recipe!

Items you need:
- Salt: a pinch
- Cilantro, chopped: 2 T
- Vine-ripened tomato, diced: 1 small
- Lime essential oil: 3 drops
- Lemon essential oil: 2 drops
- Garlic, crushed: 2 cloves
- Red onion, chopped: 1 Cup
- Avocados, mashed: 2 large
- Mixing bowl: 1

How to make it:
- Place the avocado, red onion, essential oil drops, tomatoes, cilantro, garlic, and salt into the mixing bowl
- Mix together the ingredients until well combined
- Serve with chips or fresh vegetables!

Essential Oil and Herb Salad Dressing

Who needs a boring salad when you can add a flavorful, healthy dressing?! Just put this dressing onto your favorite salad mixture and enjoy. The essential oils will give a lovely scent and healthy boost that will also keep you full after eating a salad with this dressing.

Items you need:
- Salt: a pinch
- Black pepper: a pinch
- Red wine vinegar: 3 T
- Tarragon essential oil: 3 drops
- Dijon mustard: 1 t
- Sugar: 2 t
- Olive oil: 2 T
- Mixing bowl: 1

How to make it:
- Place the sugar, essential oil drops, mustard, salt, pepper, olive oil, and red wine vinegar into the mixing bowl
- Whisk the bowl of ingredients together rapidly to emulsify the oil with the other dressing ingredients
- Pour the dressing over a bed of lettuce or spinach with your favorite salad toppings

---

Essential Oil Mexi-pie

Make dinner for the whole family with this recipe that will be sure to please! The savory essential oils used in this recipe bring a lot of flavor and pair well with the rest of the ingredients.

Items you need:
- Cheddar cheese, shredded: 2 Cups

- Black pepper essential oil: 3 drops
- Coriander essential oil: 2 drops
- Oregano essential oil: 2 drops
- Whole milk yogurt, plain: 2 Cups
- Eggs: 2
- Cilantro, dried: 1.5 t
- Baking soda: 1 t
- Baking powder: 1 T
- Flour: 1 Cup
- Cornmeal: 1.5 Cups
- Paprika: 0.25 t
- Cayenne pepper, ground: 0.5 t
- Cumin: 1 t
- Salsa: 1 Cup
- Red Bell pepper, diced: 1 medium
- Garlic, minced: 2 t
- Yellow onion, diced: 1 small
- Ground beef: 2 lbs.
- 9x13 inch baking pan: 1
- Non-stick cooking spray
- Skillet: 1
- Mixing bowl: 2

How to make it:
- Make sure your oven is heating to 375 degrees Fahrenheit
- Spray the baking pan with an even coat of non-stick spray
- Place the uncooked ground beef, bell pepper, garlic, and onion into the skillet and cook and stir until the ground beef is cooked thoroughly
- Add the paprika, cumin, cilantro, cayenne, and salsa to the skillet with cooked beef and set to a medium-low heat setting to simmer
- In one of the mixing bowls, mix together the cornmeal, baking soda, baking powder, sugar, and flour

- In the other mixing bowl, beat the eggs and yogurt together with a whisk and then stir it into the bowl of dry ingredients
- Remove the simmering skillet from the heat and stir in the essential oil drops and cheddar cheese
- Pour the beef and cheese mixture into the greased pan and top evenly with the yogurt and cornmeal mixture
- Place the filled pan into the heated oven for 30 minutes to bake
- Remove the cooked dish from the oven and serve while warm

Ginger Essential Oil Cookies

This spice-filled cookie are chewy and delicious! The essential oils add even more flavor for you to enjoy with guests and family!

Items you need:
- Sugar, coarse: 1 T
- Salt: 1 t
- Baking soda: 4 t
- Flour: 4 Cups
- Ginger essential oil: 4 drops
- Clove essential oil: 2 drops
- Cinnamon essential oil: 2 drops
- Molasses: 0.5 Cups
- Eggs: 2
- Sugar: 2 Cups
- Butter: 1.5 Cups
- Mixing bowl: 2
- Cookie sheet: 1

How to make it:
- Place the sugar and butter into the mixing bowl and cream together until fluffy

- Stir in the molasses and eggs to the creamed mixture, and then stir in the essential oil drops until completely combined
- In the other bowl, add the salt, baking soda, and flour and stir together
- Add the bowl of dry ingredients into the bowl of wet ingredients and mix them together
- Place the bowl of ingredients into the fridge for 1 hour to chill
- Make sure your oven is heating to 350 degrees Fahrenheit
- Take the bowl of cookie dough out of the fridge and form 1-inch balls out of it
- Place each ball of dough onto the baking sheet and place into the heated oven to cook for 10-12 minutes
- Take out the cookies from the oven and let them sit for a few minutes before taking them off of the sheet to serve

---

Peppermint Essential Oil Mocha

Are you craving one of your favorite holiday drinks? Even if it is that time of year, you will not find anything like this recipe at a normal coffee shop. The essential oils give it a boost of flavor and nourishment that is satisfying and delicious!

Items you need:
- Peppermint essential oil: 3 drops
- Sugar: 0.25 Cups
- Cocoa powder: 2 T
- Coffee, freshly brewed: 2 Cups
- Almond milk: 2 Cups (may also use a different milk of choice)
- Saucepan: 1
- Mixing bowl: 1

How to make it:
* Pour the milk into the saucepan and it heat while stirring until it starts to bubble
* Add the coffee into the saucepan with heated milk and turn the heat down
* Stir the cocoa powder and sugar together in the mixing bowl and then mix this into the milk and coffee
* Whisk the saucepan of ingredients until all clumps have dissolved and the liquid is thick and creamy
* Pour the saucepan liquid into 2 mugs and add 1 drop of the peppermint essential oil to each
* Stir before serving

Chai Spiced Latte with Essential Oils

Another favorite drink with even more of a flavor boost! The essential oils in this recipe add a flowery fragrance to this drink, as well as an unparalleled flavor that cannot simply be bought.

Items you need:
* Cardamom essential oil: 2 drops
* Ginger essential oil: 1 drop
* Lemongrass essential oil: 1 drop
* Milk: 0.25 Cups
* Chai tea, brewed: 0.75 Cup

How to make it:
* Pour the milk into a mug and heat in the microwave for about 10 seconds
* Remove the milk from the microwave and stir in the brewed tea
* Add the essential oil drops to the filled mug and stir
* Serve while hot

Essential Oil Pumpkin Spice Bread

Pumpkin bread is so easy and fun to make! This recipe will make a delicious pumpkin bread that adds even more delicious spice flavors with the addition of essential oils. Get ready to crave this bread as soon as it's gone!

Items you need:
* Lemon essential oil: 4 drops
* Ginger essential oil: 1 drops
* Nutmeg essential oil: 2 drops
* Clove essential oil: 2 drops
* Cinnamon essential oil: 2 drops
* Yogurt, plain: 1 Cup
* Water: 0.3 cups
* Eggs: 4
* Pumpkin puree: 1 15-oz. can
* Butter, softened: 0.5 Cups
* Coconut oil: 0.5 Cups
* Sugar: 2.75 Cups
* Baking powder: 1 t
* Baking soda: 2 t
* Salt: 1 t
* Flour: 3.5 Cups
* Mini-loaf pans: 8
* Non-stick spray
* Mixing bowl: 1

How to make it:
* Make sure your oven is heating to 325 degrees Fahrenheit
* Coat your loaf pans evenly with non-stick spray
* Place the essential oil drops, eggs, butter, coconut oil, yogurt, water, and pumpkin into one of the mixing bowls and whisk until well blended
* While whisking continuously, slowly add in the flour, salt, sugar, baking powder, and baking soda until well

combined and a fluffy batter has formed. Be sure to
scrape the sides of the bowl occasionally
- Pour an even amount of the dough into each loaf pan
  and place them into the heated oven
- Allow the pumpkin bread to bake for 35-40 minutes or
  until a toothpick stuck in the center comes out clean
- Remove the loaf pans from the oven and allow to cool
  before cutting and serving

Essential oils are a wonderful ingredient for cooking, and the
possibilities are endless! After reviewing this chapter, you
have gotten a sense of what is possible with essential oil
cooking. Not only does it help nourish our bodies, but also
helps to add flavor and variety to our meals.

Conclusion

Thank you for making it through to the end of *Essential Oil Recipes: Enhance Your Health, Beauty, and Home*, let's hope it was informative and able to provide you with all of the tools you need to achieve your goals, whatever they may be.

The next step is to use these recipes in your everyday life! There are numerous recipes for you to try that have been provided in this book that will fit into any lifestyle.

You can now feel free to improve your beauty regimen, home, and health with these essential oil recipes, as well as find some creative gift ideas for all to enjoy! Essential oils can enhance any occasion, which you have now experienced firsthand.

This book can be useful for anyone and is intended to assist you in improving your overall lifestyle. Essential oils are full of health benefits that can improve your life and even make those around you happy. Fill your home with essential oil diffusers for favorite aromas or add them to your favorite foods for a boost of nourishment. No matter the utilization, essential oils will brighten up anyone's day and help you to lead a long, healthy life.

Finally, if you found this book useful in anyway, a review on Amazon is always appreciated!